How To Maintain Your Beauty And Fitness Looking Younger

OrangeBooks Publication

Smriti Nagar, Bhilai, Chhattisgarh - 490020

Website: **www.orangebooks.in**

First Edition, 2021

ISBN: 978-93-92878-86-2

How To Maintain Your Beauty And Fitness Looking Younger

•

Sher Singh

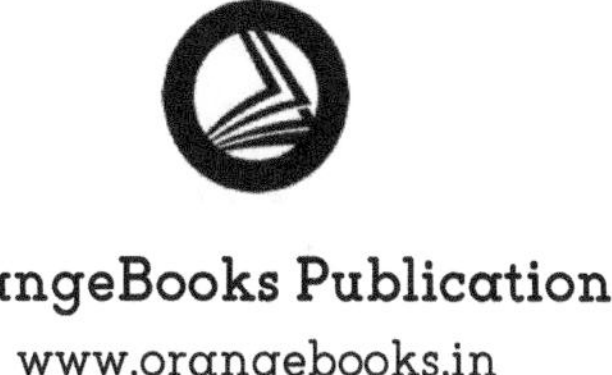

OrangeBooks Publication

www.orangebooks.in

Table of Contents

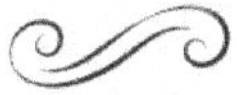

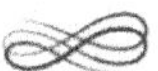

How To Maintain Your Beauty And Fitness Looking Younger

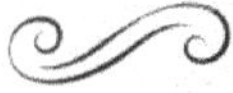

Your face is frequently one of the first things that people pay attention to you and is the focal point every time you interact with others. But as we get older, our skin changes, and we may not feel confident with our faces. Having a young face (ER) that looks and shining skin can also be a sign of health and vitality and influence how other people react to us. By practicing good skincare, modifying your lifestyle, and considering medical care, you can make your face look younger and shine; you are young, skin.

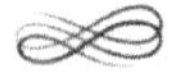

Natural Ways To Keep Teenage Skin And Shine

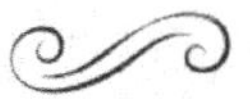

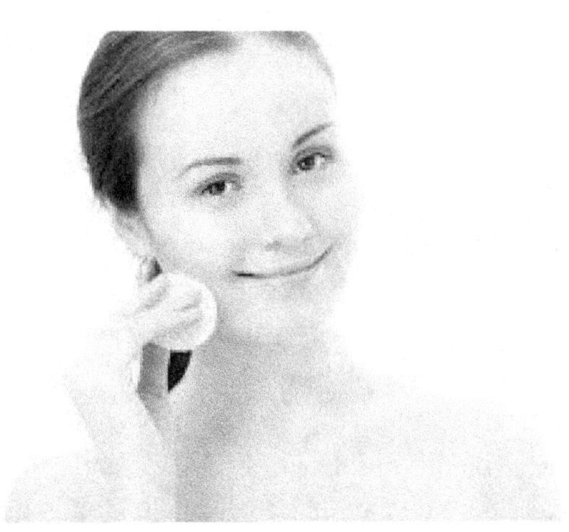

When it comes to the aspirations of skincare, the term "shining" seems to be at the top of everyone's list. So, to look for the best recommendations for healthy and beautiful skin, we comb the literature, talk to experts, and turn to the ritual-tested time: only items that work with capital are included in this list. -W. Here are 24 tried-and-true strategies to keep your skin glowing:

1.   Use Mineral-Based Sunscreen Every Day.

Every day, throughout the year, SPF is clean; mineral-based must be used. "Ultraviolet radiation is a firm carcinogenic," said Heidi Waldorf, M.D., Certified Council Dermatologist. "If you don't care, consider Ray Vanity-UV is the main cause of skin aging texture and color changes," Waldorf suggested using SPF 30 or mineral-based sunscreen (looking for active ingredients such as zinc oxide or titanium dioxide) as a final step in your morning skincare routine to protect your skin. Mineral sunscreen should be used as the last step before applying makeup because it is a physical barrier: Every skincare activity that you are trying to apply after not penetrating.

Besides that - smart sun care goes far out of SPF. Always be careful with how much time you spend in the sun (read: Don't sunbathe for sports) and wear hats and other protective clothes.

2.   Try Completing Collagen. A *

Your body's most abundant protein - and your skin - collagen. And, unfortunately, our natural reserves of essential protein spend with age. Collagen supplements contain amino acids, which have been shown to promote our nail hair, skin, and health. By swallowing hydrolyzed collagen peptides, supplements are absorbed by the body and can then support natural collagen levels by stimulating our cell fibroblasts (or what makes collagen and elastin in the first place), thus promoting healthy, luminous, and strong skin. This is supported by cold hard data, too: This collagen peptide has been shown in the study to help skin elasticity, hydration, and dermal collagen density. Look at the list of collagen supplements for us for our personal advice.

3.   Exfoliation.

"I do not recommend scrubs or hard cloth," explained Nancy Samolitis, certified dermatologist, M.D., which includes peeling the skin as one of the top tips for shining skin. "Exfoliation of light, with nonirritective acid cleaners or toner that dissolves dead skin cells on the surface, [will] cause the skin to shine." How? Releasing the outer layer of excessive dead skin cells will help soften the skin texture, increase the absorption rate of your skincare products, and brighten your skin.

4.   Take Care Of Your Intestine.

Research shows that the underlying intestinal health problems can manifest on the skin in many ways, from stains to turning red. The connection even has a name: skin-gut axis. Overall intestinal health is nuanced and complex and important (for so, so many reasons) for everyone to take the time to learn how to care for and feed your own unique intestinal flora. However, for the motive of this article, this is a general guideline: anything that is unhealthy for your intestines (i.e., sugar, processed foods) can cause microbial imbalances and trigger oxidative stress and inflammatory processes, not only in the intestine but throughout the body. Over time, it is left unchecked; this imbalance can also manifest as a skin problem. See also: This is why you have to heal your intestines if you want clear skin.

5.   Increase The Amount Of Healthful Fat In Your Diet.

"Healthy fats like those found in almonds, flaxseed, and avocados can help your body create healthy and robust cell membranes, [which] can protect against environmental harm by maintaining the skin barrier," Samolitis explained. "Not eating enough healthy fats can cause skin and hair to dry," Waldorf says, adding that "increasing these fats in a diet can aid in specific skin diseases characterized by extreme drought." Salmon, chia seeds, olive oil, & whole eggs are some more nutritious meals that should be known for glowing skin.

6.   Maintain Healthy Skin Microbiomas.

Healthy and balanced skin microbiomes are as important as healthy and balanced intestinal microbiomas to keep the skin healthy and balanced. This minuscule microorganism keeps hydrated skin and chewy against free radicals, protects against external aggressors, and even provides protection from UV light damage. Avoid strong soap and scrub, which can remove vital oil and microorganisms that make up skin microbiomas to maintain your balance. Use skincare products designed to support healthy skin microbiomes, such as those containing pre-, pro-and postbiotics (here's the list of our best products to support healthy skin microbiomas).

7. Immediately After Bathing, Apply Skincare Products.

Maybe one of the most important components of healthy skin is moisture. In addition to quality skincare routines, the time you apply your product can affect moisture retention. Tip Top Waldorf: Pay attention to your skincare routine as soon as you jump out of the bathroom. "Apply the moisturizer every day on the face and body after washing, filling, and sealing in moisture," he said. "Much better keep the skin good rather than trying to catch up after the skin is dry, inflamed, and uncomfortable."

8. Follow A Face Massage Regimen.

Not only does face massage feel good, but it also helps to relieve tension and promote circulation, which helps to maintain skin cells healthy and aids lymphatic drainage. Use a jade roller or commit to a daily face gua sha program. It simply takes a few minutes a day and the glow you'll get from the facial massage (thanks to the enhanced circulation) will be well worth it.

9. Consume Meals That Are High In Antioxidants.

"The more vibrant, the better," explains Samolitis. "Dark, leafy greens and berries are my favorites." Fruits and vegetables are, without indecision, the most abundant sources of antioxidants. Blueberries, kale, spinach, and—bonus—dark chocolate are among antioxidant-rich foods to add to your diet.

10. Stay Active.

Sports increase blood flow throughout the body so that it carries vital oxygen, nutrition, and minerals to the skin. In essence: exercise causes brighter skin and looks better.

11. Use Vitamin C.

One of the best topical materials for shining, plain and simple skin is vitamin C - which works on all skin types to level and enlightens the tone. Research to reserve these claims is the voice and broad: Vitamin C can promote balanced pigmentation, protect against environmental aggressors, brighten the skin tone, and promote collagen and elastin production.

12. Don't Choose Your Skin.

As a general rule, after your product is applied, keep your hand (most likely dirty) from your face. "Choose skin-acne, infection, or just itchy area - causing the worsening problem and in the end, it can [lead to] infections and scars," Waldorf said.

13. Stay Hydrated.

This is not a myth: drinking enough water for overall skin health. Stay adequately hydrated makes your skin moisturized, healthy, and, you guessed it, shine. It's not to mention all other endless benefits from drinking enough H20. While eight (8 ounces) glasses per day are general guidelines, water intake instead of one-size-fitting so listens to what your body needs.

14.   Use An Alternative Retinoid Or Retinol.

"Is your skin better with over-the-counter retinol or retinoid strength of recipes? This material is on my list to promote healthy and radiant skin," said Samolitis. "First, it really represents DNA damage from the sun and the environment and can even protect against Prizenker skin lesions. Second, it makes the top layer of the skin from building and looks boring by promoting accelerated skin cell turnover."

15.   Get Ordinary Facials.

We know, we know - this is not always worth it. But if it's in your budget, getting an ordinary facial is one of the best ways to maintain a healthy and radiant Visage, said Samolitis. You are ideally aiming for one face per month, which falls in time with the natural update cycle of your skin cells.

16.   Avoid Potentially Annoying Foods.

You already know what it is: packaged food, processed, and high sugar, as well as milk. "Excess sugar, milk, and processed food can cause the inflammatory process on the skin, which leads to breakouts," Samolitis said if you can only commit to removing one of the food without - for processed sugar because the latest research has confirmed the relationship between high sugar food and acne, and head-to-to-to-to-toe inflammation problems.

17. Don't Smoke.

Obviously, but because of so many reasons, it is worth maintaining: smoking has a detrimental effect on your body from head to leg. While the light is worried, "smoking limits the supply of oxygen to the skin, increasing the accumulation of damaging free radicals and increasing the risk of some skin cancer," Waldorf explained.

18. Pamper Facial Masks.

In our opinion, facial masks don't even be considered indulgent - you have to apply them regularly. To maximize light, choose hyaluronic mask materials such as hyaluronic acid, sodium hyaluronate, and vitamin E.

19. Strengthen your skin barrier.

Dry skin, fragments, dries? Your skin barrier is likely to be compromised. Strengthen it by using moisturizers and cleaners formulated by ceramide, an important component of the skin barrier (which can be stripped of things like over-cleansing).

20. Get Your Beauty Sleep.

But other important reasons for prioritizing sleep: sleeping inadequate or disturbed can bring havoc on your skin. Research has shown that poor sleep grades can contribute to the increase in signs of skin aging (fine lines and wrinkles) and compromised skin barrier function. As with water, eight hours are standard practical rules for sleeping, but always listening to your body.

21. Keep Your Makeup-And Makeup Tool - Clean.

The makeup brush, bag, and sponge are basically a breeding place for bacterial proliferation, dead skin cells, oil, and dirt - all of which can seriously inhibit your search for shining skin. So, save sanitary goods! Clean your makeup tool regularly, ideally every week.

22. Keep Things Lukewarm.

One of the most common facial washing errors: using the wrong water temperature. Rinse your skin (and hair) with water that is too hot can strip the natural oil skin barrier, which can dry the skin and cause a compromised barrier. Water that is too cold will not finish work and may leave dirt and makeup on your skin. So when it comes to cleaning, stay at a water temperature that is lukewarm.

23. Minimize Stress.

It is easier to say than done, we know, but the feeling of chronic stress can seriously damage your skin - and even trigger a number of problems, including the autoimmune path. Moreover, the reason for the right self-care routine, whatever might look for you (although maybe we suggest some of the tips mentioned above, like taking the time for facial, facials, sports, and sleeping beauty masks).

24. Moisturize.

Need more to say? Moisturizing the skin is one of the fastest tickets to shiny coat. Don't waste your daily moisturizer, even if you have naturally oily skin. Also, invest in proven hydration ingredients (peptides, electrolytes, ceramides, etc.).

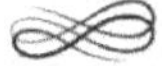

Benefits Of Beauty Training

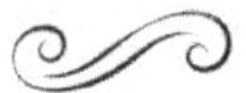

There are many reasons to exercise. For some people, it's because you book a beach vacation, while others focus on staying healthy. Whatever your incentive, we can all agree that the advantages of exercise are undeniable. But there are results that are quiet: healthy skin. Read on to learn more about the rewards of skin and beauty that come from sweat regularly

➤ **Instant Glow.**

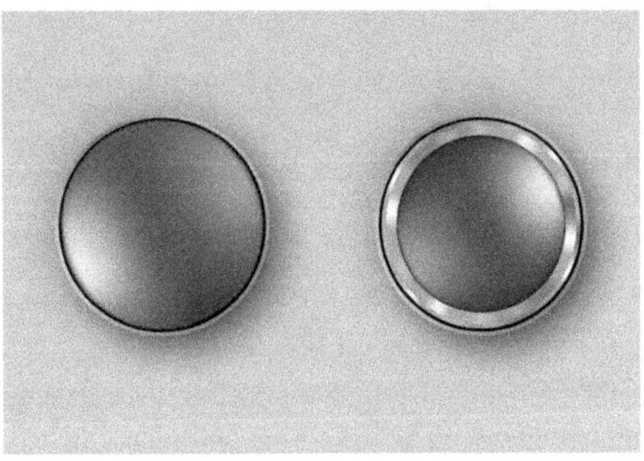

When you pump your heart from aerobic exercise, you supply your skin with oxygenated blood doses, said Noëlle S. Sherber, M.D., a Certified Dermatologist board based in Baltimore, Maryland. "This gives you a good post-practice light."

➢ Wrinkle Reduction.

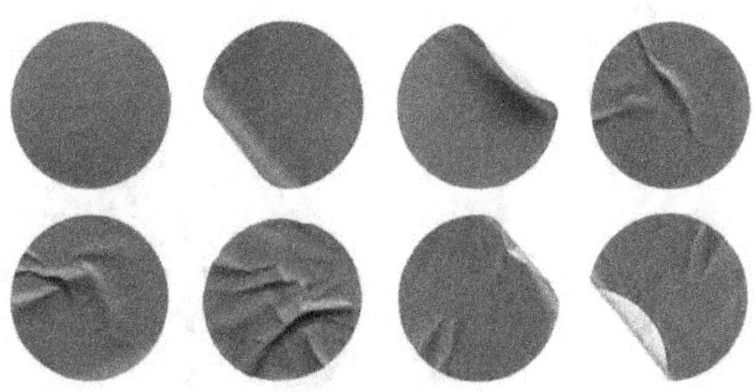

Exercise also helps maintain a healthy level of hormone cortisol related to stress, said Sherber. "High cortisol levels are associated with an increase in sebum production, which means more acne," he said. Too much cortisol can also cause the collagen in damaged skin, said Sherber, which can increase wrinkles and slack. "The exercise actually supports collagen production," said Amy Dixon, physiology and celebrity coach based in Los Angeles. "The urge in this protein helps keep your skin strong, springy, and elastic."

> ## Acne Help.

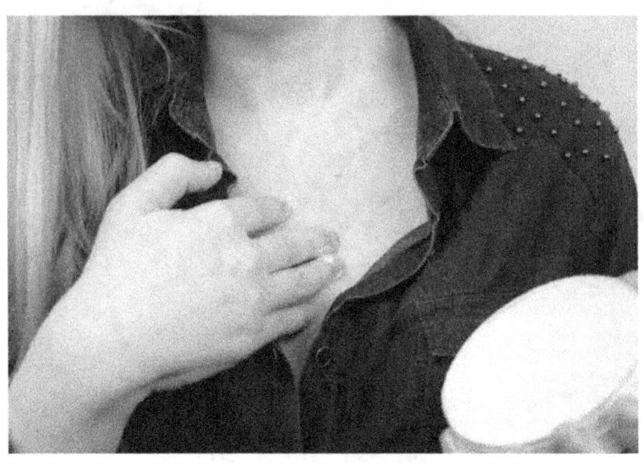

Regular exercise increases circulation. "It maintains your skin, carrying more blood flow and oxygen for it," said Mauro C. Romita, M.D., a certified plastic surgeon and founder of the June Center for Beauty Synergy in New York City. "This will help draw poisons from the body." Plus, all those who sweat clean solid skin pores. "Exercising corrects hormonal imbalances that can cause adult zits," Romita said.

To reap the effects of the beneficial skin from exercise, some additional steps are needed, Sherber warns. "If you are prone to pimples, make sure to keep the soft cleaning wipes and aroma-free in your gym bag." Be sure to clean the face and other areas that tend to come out immediately after exercising, he said. "For eczema, wear a cloth that makes sweat from the skin because the dry-dry-dry cycle will dry your skin and fishing flares," Sherber said. And especially, avoid exercising with makeup on your face.

➢ Healthier Hair.

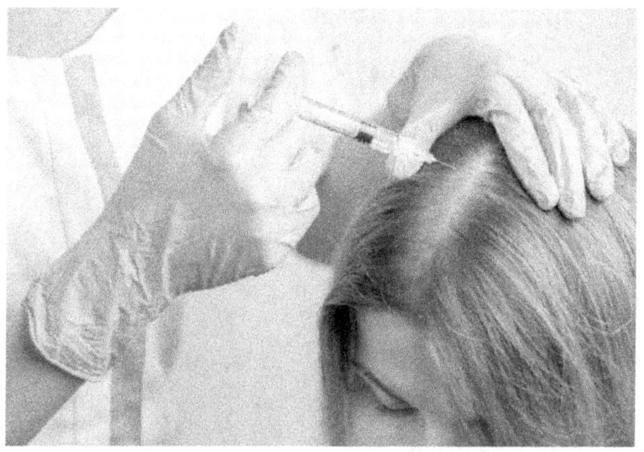

Enhanced blood flow helps keep your hair stronger and healthier, said Dixon. This blood, full of nutrition, stimulates hair follicles and promotes growth. "Exercise is also a big stress relief," he said. "Lower stress means your hair tends to be fragile and, worse, fall out." Even if you are as free of stress as cucumber, Dixon recommends checking with your dermatologist about hair loss to override other causes.

As for the best type of exercise for your skin, Dixon says it's all good. "Every modality will increase circulation and reduce stress," he said, "but it's a wise step to mix your practice as often as possible." Try adding 30 minutes from some simple yoga postures or walking fast to your day three times a week, said Dixon, to see beauty back in your hair and skin.

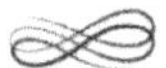

Ways To Enhance Your Beauty Naturally

❖ Drink Plenty Of Water To Save Your Body Hydrated.

Don't turn your eyes. Maybe you know this will happen, but it must be said. Dehydration makes wrinkles more clear and makes your body from doing things to do.

Drink water slowly all day, every day, and it will help improve your beauty. If you try to compensate by drinking one gallon of water after dinner, you won't absorb everything (and you have to get up to go piss when you have to get your beauty sleep!).

❖ Clean Your Body In With Water

Suppose you drink drinks that make you dehydrated, such as coffee and alcohol, hydrate before and after to eliminate effects. If you like your morning coffee, I'm not saying you have to give up. You brew you! But challenging yourself to drink a glass of first water in the morning, and then reward yourself with your Joe.

The body uses water to clean. If we can't water them out that way, they build somewhere else or appear on our skin.

❖ Regular Exercises For Healthy Bodies.

About 20% of the body's elimination happens through sweat. Keep things circulating by sweat? Sit in a sauna, sport, or do both!

Bikram yoga, cycling, or going jogging is a great way to work until sweating. Is it suitable for you! Be sure to wash your face before working outside, especially if you use make-up. When you sweat, your pores are open, and you invite anything around to come to gather. Aka-you makeup, dirt, and other remnants of your day. To avoid reabsorbing all you just sweated out, shower promptly after your workout.

Exercise also releases endorphins, and we know to be happy, your brand is much more beautiful! Plus, getting your heartbeat up will give your cheek some colors while keeping your heart healthy.

❖ Brew Self-Bath With Teapot.

We are water-themed enough so far. But that's how we pop in the world do it!

Bathing is a relaxing uber, relieving stress that uses on all your existence, including your skin.

Your shower to the next level with a large brewing, strong (I like which this happens) Teapot tea and add it to the water. Of course, make sure the water is not too hot before you jump (is this disclaimer needed?).

Try the following tea in your bathroom. In this way, you can like the benefits of plants from head to toe!

- Chamomile for skin smoothness
- Echinacea to increase skin hydration
- Fennel for Vitamin Rich sources
- Yarrow to clog the cleaning pore
- Coffee rejuvenates your skin

❖ Keep An Eye On Sulfur As A Mineral Beauty.

Overall, eating nutritious food promotes good health and good skin, but there are some nutrients that are mainly beautiful.

Sulfur, although it is not usually included in the nutritional label or is considered an important nutrient, is the fourth most abundant mineral in the body and is very important for many processes. Your hair and skin will be soft and smooth if you have enough sulfur in your body. Sulfur can be found in eggs, plants including broccoli and cabbage, and radish.

Zinc is another ore that will make you more beautiful and interesting. Get your zinc from seeds like pumpkin, poppy, or sunflower seeds, spirulina, or shellfish.

❖ Be Makeup-Free - Get Naked.

Will makeup-less one day a week will give your pores the opportunity to breathe.

If you go without makeup, it doesn't sound fun for you; make sure you use mineral makeup so that your skin doesn't absorb toxic chemicals.

❖ Orange You Glad You Read This?

Dark orange foods high in beta carotene may actually warm your skin. Sweet potatoes and butternut squash thrive in the winter. Carrots, peaches, and apricots are also terrific options.

Because vitamin A is fat-soluble, take some healthy fat at the same time to get the most out of it. After drinking carrot juice, eat a slice of avocado or spray some olive oil over a baked sweet potato.

❖ Whiten Your Teeth Using Charcoal Powder.

You can use this dark powder as a dental whitening treatment. Add to your toothpaste or place it directly on your toothbrush (do this above the sink to avoid chaos). This treatment, several times a week, will draw dirt from the mouth and lift the stains from your teeth for a whiter smile!

❖ Coloring Your Hair With Herbs.

If you are looking for ways to lighten your hair naturally or add a little color, hair rinses are easy to make and can be used regularly to maintain your scalp, soften, and add fine colors to your hair. For tea, let it cool, then rinse your hair with shampoo.

Leave for 20 minutes and conditions as usual. Try the best herbs for dyeing hair:

- Black tea or coffee to grow color and add a smooth reddish tone.
- Chamomile relieves hair and soothes the scalp.

- Rosemary cleans hair.

Maybe adding extra steps to your bath routine doesn't sound too interesting. You might also simply add some components to your shampoo. To deepen the color of your dark hair, use cocoa powder and cinnamon in your shampoo.

❖ Eyebrow Treatment Tips - Don't Ignore This.

We conditioned our hair but mercilessly ignored our eyelashes. What's wrong with it? We are here to promote equality for all hair.

Slide oil soft or organic eye cream at the end of your eyelashes and above your eyebrows at night to keep them soft. It's very important if you haven't turned to a natural mascara!

Be sure to keep your eyebrows well-formed to frame your face. If you revoke, it is not your specialty; try waxing or threading to keep it beautiful.

❖ Every Woman Wants Bigger Breasts.

According to the beauty basically, one of our favorites by Brigitte Mars, the French woman has long used hydrotherapy to promote cheerful breasts. To increase circulation, end the shower with 30 seconds of cold water.

Increased circulation can help maintain Breast Company. You can also change between hot and cold. In a 30-second increase, it ends coldly for extra circulation.

❖ How To Keep Positive Thoughts.

Thinking of good thoughts and keeping positive thoughts and intentions will really make you more beautiful. Sadness wears us physically and emotionally. Cheer up by surrounding yourself with beautiful things using the following methods:

- Keep the flower vase in your room,

- Mix delicious and relaxed aroma like neroli throughout your house, and

- Decorate your home in decorations that inspire and please you.

- Make sure your room is clean to prevent confusion and trouble, and

- Notice how the food you eat makes you feel.

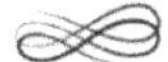

How To Stay Suitable Forever: Tips To Save Moving When Life Comes In.

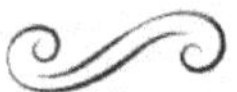

> ### One Work Why Not Only Works Out.

Our reason for starting exercises is very important for whether we will stay up, said Michelle fresh, director of the University of Michigan Sport, Health and research activities and policy centers. Too often, "the community promotes sports and fitness by linking to short-term motivation, guilt, and shame." There is some evidence, he said, that young people will go to the gym more if their reasons are appearance-based, but our early 20s are not a lot of fuel motivation. Also unclear or future aid destination ("I want to get a suit, I want to lose weight"). Fresh, Author No Sweat: How simple motivational science brings your lifetime fitness, saying we will be more successful if we focus on direct positive feelings such as stress reduction, increased energy, and making friends. "The only way we will prioritize for practice is if it will provide some kind of really interesting and valuable benefits for everyday life," he said.

➢ Two Down To A Slow Start.

The danger of a typical new year resolution approach to fitness, said personal coach Matt Roberts, is that people "jump and do everything - change their diet, start exercising, stop drinking and smoking - and in a few weeks, they have motivations that are missing or getting too tired. If you are not yet in shape, it will take time. " He likes high intensity (HIIT) interval trends and encourages people including some, "but to do that every day will be too strong for most people." Do it once (or twice, most) a week, combined with slow jogs, swimming, and fast walking - plus two or three days of rest, at least for the first month. "It will give someone the opportunity to have a high-intensity training session."

➢ You Do Not Have To Like It.

It's helpful to not try to make yourself do the things that actively you do not like, said Segar, who suggested thinking about the kinds of activities - roller-skating? Riding a bicycle? - You love as a child. But do not feel you have to really enjoy the sport. "Many people hold on sport said: 'I feel better when I do it.'" There are elements that might be fun, like your body's physical response and the feeling grew stronger and the pleasure that comes with mastering the sport.

"For many people, the obvious choice is not that they will enjoy," said Sniehotta, who is also director of the Unit for Policy Research National Institute for Health in the Behavioral Sciences, "so they have to look beyond them. It may be sports or simple things that are different, like sharing activities with others. "

➢ Be Kind To Yourself.

Individual motivation - or lack of it - is just part of the bigger picture. Money, the demands of parenting, or even where you live all can become a stumbling block, said Sniehotta. Physical activity might be influenced by fatigue, melancholy, stress from poor workers or family members. "It will be simpler to maintain physical exercise if you have a lot of support around you," he stated. "You may feel more at ease conducting outdoor physical activity in certain sections of the country than in others. It was problematic to conclude that persons who do not have adequate physical activity lack motivation."

Fresh suggest being realistic. "Skip ideal to go to the gym five days a week. Be careful with the job requirements and the related family when you start because if you organize yourself with goals that are too big, you will fail, and you will feel like a failure. At the end of the week, I always ask my clients to reflect on what worked and what did not. It may be suitable for a walk at lunch, but you do not have the energy after work to do. "

➢ Do Not Rely On A Whim.

"If you want the willpower to do something, you do not really want to do it," said Segar. Instead, think of sports "in terms of why we are doing and what we want to get from physical activity. How can I benefit today? How do I feel when I move? How do I feel after I move?"

➢ Find Destination.

Anything that allows you to exercise when beating another goal would help, said Sniehotta. "It gives you more satisfaction, and higher costs do not." For example, walking or cycling to work or friends by joining a health club, or running with a friend. "Our goal is to spend more time in the countryside and run to help you do that."

Try to combine physical pursuit with something else. "For example, in my work, I do not use the lift, and I tried to reduce the email, so when possible, I run into people," said Sniehotta. "During the day, I walked into the office, I had a lot of moving around the building, and I really get around 15,000 steps. Try to make physical activity as much as possible to hit meaningful targets."

➢ Make A Habit.

When you run, it can be tiring just out the door - where are your shoes? Your water bottle? What route would you take? After a while, showing sniehottta, "There is no cost associated with the event." Doing regular physical activity and planning for it "helps make sustainable behavior." Sessions are missing not.

➢ Make A Strategy And Set Goals.

What if you are unable to exercise due to a lack of time? This is absolutely true for many people who have two jobs or have a lot of responsibilities, but is it true for you? This might be a priority problem, Sniehotta said. "The first is 'action planning,' where you plan where, when, and how you'll do it and strive to keep doing it," he says. The second type is 'Koping Planning': "Anticipating things that can block and place a plan to become a place for motivation again." Freshly added: "Most people do not give themselves permission to prioritize self-care behavior such as sports."

➢ Save Short And Sharp.

Practice does not need to take an hour, said Roberts. "Well, structured 15-minute exercise can be very effective if you are really pressed for time." As for a longer session, he said: "You tell yourself that you will take the time and change your schedule accordingly."

➢ Ten If It Doesn't Work Change It.

Rain for a week, you don't run once, and then you feel guilty. "This is a combination of emotions and lack of confidence that brings us to the point where, if people fail several times, they think it is the failure of the entire project," said Sniehotta. Remember, it's possible to go back to the track.

If the previous training regime has not been successful, do not blame yourself or try it again - just try something else, he said. "We have the mentality that if you can't reduce weight, it's your fault." If you can, though, modify it by: 'This method doesn't work for me, let's try something different,' there is a more likely For you, and it prevents you from blaming yourself, who doesn't help. "

➢ Add Resistance And Balance Of Training As We Get Older.

"We began to lose muscle mass over around 30," Hollie Grant said, personal training and Pilates instructors and the owner of Pilates. Resistance training (using weight, such as pedestrians, or equipment, such as resistance ribbons) is important, and he said: "This will help keep muscle mass or at least slow losses. There wants to be some form of aerobic exercise, and we will also recommend people start adding The challenge of balance because our balance is affected with age. "

➢ Up Ante.

"If you do 5rb running and you don't know whether you have to push it faster or go further, rank your activities from one to 10," Grant said. "As you see the numbers down, it's just starting to push yourself a little faster," Roberts said that, with regular exercise, you must see progress for a period of two weeks and push yourself if you feel easier. "You're looking for a change in speed or durability or your strength."

➤ Exercise From Home.

If you have attentive responsibility, Roberts says you can do many things in a small area at home. "In the living room, it's easy to do the routine where you might alternate between doing foot exercises and arm exercises," he said. "This is called peripheral heart action training. Making six or eight exercises, this effect occurs between the upper and lower body produces a strong metabolic lift of beautiful and cardiovascular exercises." Try squat, half press-up, lungs, tricep dips, and glute salaries. "You raise your heartbeat, work your muscles, and have good general exercises." It's no more than 15-20 minutes and only requires a seat for tricep dips - although dumbbells can help, too.

➤ Become Short Of Breath.

Housework and gardening are frequently touted as ways to help us meet our weekly fitness goals, but is it really that simple? "Size really is you get generally hot, breathless, and you are working at a level where, if you have a conversation with someone while you do it, you panting a little," said Roberts. "With gardening, you will have to do more heavy gardening - digging - not just weeding. If you walk the dog, you can make it a genuine exercise session - running with the dog, or find a route which includes some of the hills ".

➤ Be Wise About The Disease.

Joslyn Thompson Rule, a personal trainer, said: "The general rule is if it is above the neck - headache or runny nose - while pay attention to your feelings, you are generally OK to do some sort of exercise. If under the neck - if you have trouble breathing - the rest. The key is to be reasonable. If you are planning on doing high-intensity exercise, you will take a step down, but sometimes it just moves; it can make you feel better. " After recovering from an illness, he said, trust your instincts. "You do not want to go straight back to training four times a week. You may want to do the same number of sessions but make them shorter or do a little. "

> ## Seek Advices After Injury.

Obviously, how quickly you start exercising again depending on the type of injury, and you should seek advice from your doctor. Psychologically, though, said Thompson Rule: "Even when we do everything as it should be, there are dips in the road. It will not be a linear progression to get better. "

> ## Take It Slowly After Pregnancy.

Again, Thompson said Rule, listen to your body - and your doctor's advice on a six-week postnatal checkup you. After a cesarean section, return to the practice will be slow, while the back-related injuries and problems with pregnancy-belly muscles all affect how quickly you can get back into training and may require physiotherapy. "When you're running and have a little more energy, depending on where you were before (some women never trained before pregnancy), began the regime after the baby is quite something to do,"

Thompson said Rule. "Patience. I get added emails from women asking when they will get their stomach flat again from nothing. Temper, take care of yourself, and take care of your baby. When you are feeling a little more energetic, slowly back into your routine." He recommends starting with "things that are very basic as walking and carrying your baby [in a sling]."

➤ Tech Can Help.

For people who are goal-oriented, Grant said, it may be useful to monitor progress closely but "allow flexibility in your goals. You may have days of stress at work, go out for a run and did not do it quickly, and then think: 'I just will not bother anymore.' "However," It can start to get an addictive little bit, and then you do not listen to your body, and you are more at risk of injury. "

➤ Winter Is Not An Excuse

Winter is not always time for hibernation," Thompson said Rule. Be decisive, put your trainers by the door, and try not to think about the cold / drizzle/greyness. "It's the same as going to the gym - it was the voice in our heads that make us feel like it was a hassle, but once you are there, you think: 'Why do I procrastinate about it for so long?'"

➤ Keep Bite-Sized

I've tried and broken several times to establish a consistent running routine, but it was because I kept pushing myself too hard. Just because I can walk for an hour does not mean I have to. Running for 20-30 minutes two or three times a week has tremendously improved my fitness and made it simpler to adjust.

➢ Own Prizes

I saved a big pocket of a symbol gem in my car to motivate myself to go to the gym, let myself be a handful before practice. Sometimes I throw some wine gums for surprise elements.

➢ Calls In Reinforcements

I use extensive network fitness podcasts and online communities. On the days I don't have a drive, I will listen to the fitness podcast, and when I arrive at home, I am really determined to make the right choice. In fact, I will be happy because of it. Your brain responds very well to repetition and reinforcement, so after you make a difficult initial change, it becomes easier from time to time.

➢ Use Visual Motivations

I have saved a "star" on my calendar for the past two years. After three years, it is not chronic. I put a gold star on the days that I exercised, and it was a good visual motivator when I felt like a snail. I run, use our home cross-trainer and do a ski fitness program from the application. My better core strength has helped me run and my ability to bring my disabled child when needed.

➤ Keep The Alarm From Reach

If, like me, you want to get up early to exercise, or it doesn't happen, move your alarm clock from your bed and next to your kit. After you wake up to turn it off, you might keep going!

➤ Follow The Rules Of Four Days

I have a simple rule that can apply to any fitness activity - I do not allow more than four days passing between sessions. So, if I know I have a few busy days, I made sure I ran in front of them, so I had "bent" my four days. With the exception of the disease, injury, or family emergency, I have attached to this rule for ten years.

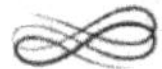

Open Skin Without Defects With These Simple Beauty Tips For The Face

Your skin is an indicator of the story about how well your feelings are inside. This is why it is very important for you to care for your skin and spoil it ridiculous from time to time. But thanks to our very busy lifestyle, regular skincare often tends to retreat. Add this problem; Constant stress, dirt, pollution, sun exposure, and our eternal love for junk food, and you can already smell extraordinary skin! But don't worry, Miss! We have something that will bring a big smile to your lips and amazing light on your face. Exceptional skin is not too difficult to be achieved honestly, as long as you are regular, determined, and diligent.

Beauty tips for this face will give you brighter and luminous skin that you will love. This beauty tip for the face has reached the test of time and exit wins. There are the basics that your skin doctor wishes you know and follow. Also, these tips have your grandmother's covenant, who is labeled in all.

It's a beauty guide for all beauty addicts and skincare out there. Try these beauty tips for the face first, and don't forget to thank you later!

1.   Wash Your Face Twice A Day.

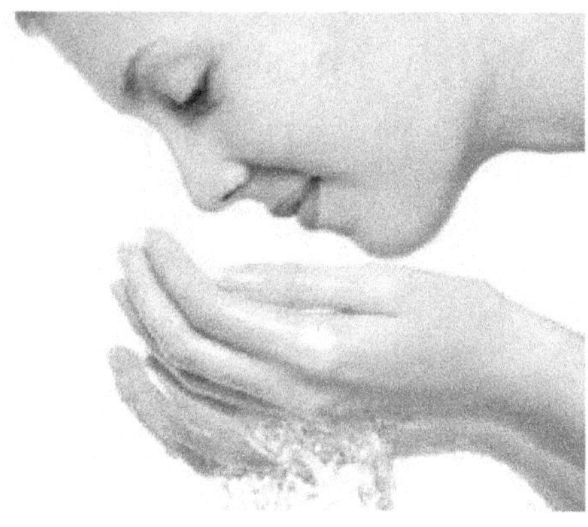

Clean or wash your face. The basic form of a good beauty routine for defective skin and shouldn't be compromised, no matter what. Wash your face helps remove dirt, dirt, and dirt and is a beauty tip that is important for the face. And by washing, we internally opposed your face with a soft foaming cleaner like a pure white anti-pollution pool + purity face washing. This face lighting is enriched with activated carbon that helps eliminate the trace of your pollution damage thoroughly makes your skin look really clean, perfect, and radiant. Using facial washing is very important because it only rinses your face with water is not enough, and more often than not, dirt and minerals in water can damage your skin and make it out.

2.   Massage Your Face.

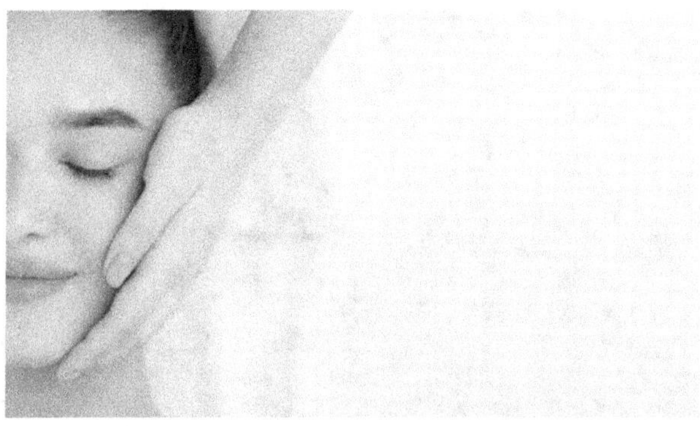

Facial massage is a general practice followed by many women as part of their beauty routine, and indeed so because there are too many benefits of facial massage. This is a natural way to relieve stress and to improve your mood. This is a surprising beauty tip for the face because it helps stimulate collagen production and blood on the skin. Regularly massaging your face tightens the skin and lifts your face muscles. This is an extraordinary anti-aging treatment and works well to give you young light. In addition, facial massage also benefits the condition of inflamed skin such as acne and rosacea. Light manipulation on the skin grows blood flow and oxygen needed for healing, plus this helps expel poisons that are often responsible for breakouts.

3.   Drink Plenty Of Water.

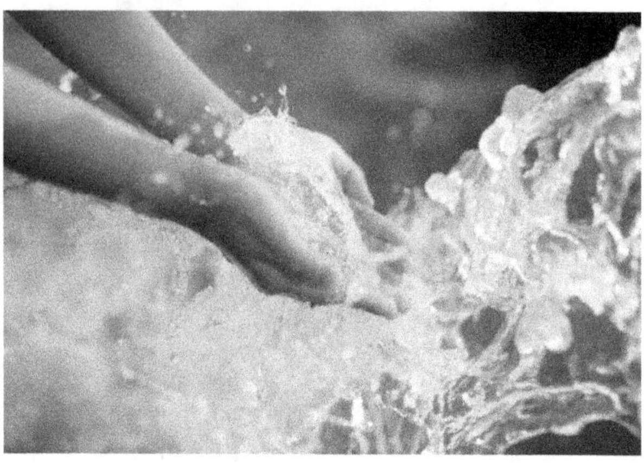

Water has many benefits of skincare and is a natural and super safe tip for flawless skin. Skin, just like your other organs, need water to function properly. If you don't drink enough water, you seize your skin with enough hydration. The lack of hydration will show your skin because it will make it look dry, tight, and scaly. Dry skin has less resilience and is more susceptible to wrinkles. When water is lost in large quantities every day, you need to replace it somehow. Water flushed poisons from our vital organs while also carrying nutrition to cells, which helps organs function at the optimal level. In connection with the skin, it is better to reduce acne, signs, and acne, even delay the aging process to a certain extent.

4.   Wear Sunscreen Every Day.

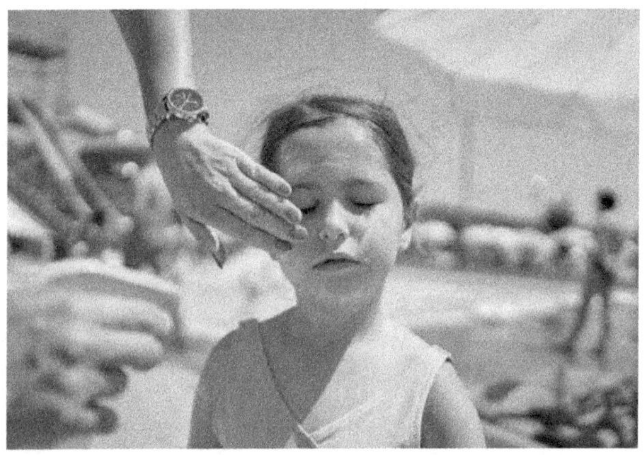

If you want healthy skin, shine, and wrinkle-free, it is important for you to follow the tip of this beauty for the face without fail every day. Although wearing sunscreen might seem like additional tasks in your beauty routine that do not show direct results, the truth is, using sunscreen every day today will definitely ensure that your skin thank you ten years later. You should never leave home without using some sunscreen to ensure that your skin suffers the minimum sun damage. Sunscreen prevents wrinkles, spots, loosens, and skin cancer. Select SPF with at least 30 PA +++, which will give you extra hydration and unmatched protection.

5. Use A Face Mask Regularly.

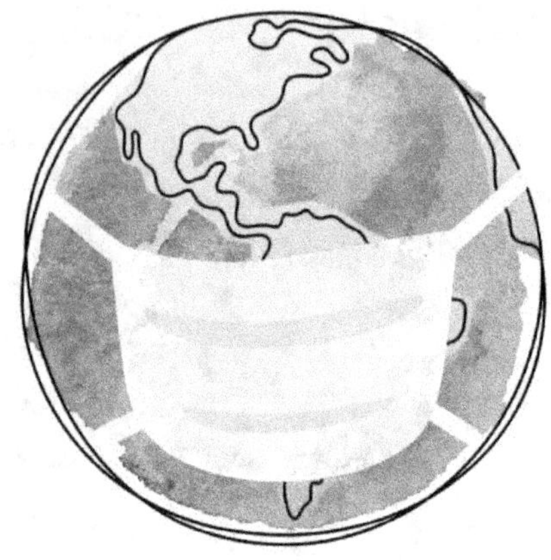

If you have to rob yourself about spoiling your face mask and pamper yourself in some Netflix and relax for the weekend, then it must have shown. If you want an easy and rapid way to reach healthy and springy skin, then you have to make your own face mask now. The benefits of using many facial masks and they are designed for different skin types, ages and solve specific problems for fast and targeted actions. If you are looking for a tip of beauty for the face at home to reach the skin without defects, then the face mask is perfect. Using the correct face mask helps to hydrate the skin, eliminate excess oil and improves the appearance of your pores. They are also the best way to help remove dirt.

6. Simply Sleep.

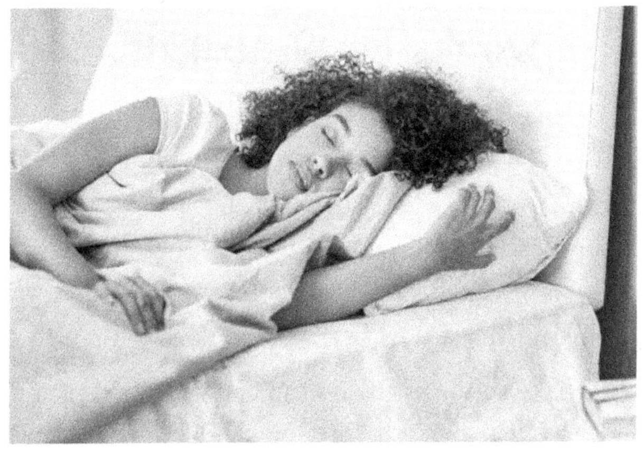

If you are tired, then it will definitely show on your face. This is why, regardless of all the fun in beauty care for your face, it is very important for you to sleep enough every night. After all, sleeping at night is called catching up sleeping for a reason! Sleep helps balance your body's hydration and keep your skin healthy and hydrated. Your body grows blood flow to the skin when you delay, which means you wake up with a healthy light. Skimp on sleep, and your skin can look drab, ashen, or lifeless. If you need to smooth out your wrinkles and fine lines, we suggest you press the sack now. But don't forget to sleep with a sleeping pillowcase and sleep on your back not to harm your skin when you sleep.

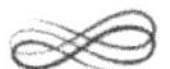

Face Beauty Tips : Dos And Don'ts For Naturally Gorgeous Skin

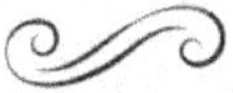

> ➢ **Golden Rules**

Do it: Make sure you always (and our intentions always) remove your makeup before the sheets. The skin needs to breathe overnight. And makeup prevents it, such as leaving it on clogging pores that can cause defects and/or blackheads. Don't have a makeup remover? Just add some olive oil on cotton pads and gently massage to your face to remove makeup and dirt.

Don't: Forget that peeling is very necessary. At least once or twice a week, peeling your skin to remove the layer of dead skin will definitely leave you with healthier, light, and brighter skin. You can also apply walnut pasta in the form of powder with yogurt to peel your skin because antioxidants present in walnuts help remove dirt and promote shining skin.

> ➢ **Sun And Skin.**

Do it: Apply sunscreen with SPF at least 15, which blocks the UVA light and UVB. Because exposure to live sunlight can cause wrinkles, age spots, and other skin problems, you must protect your skin from the sun.

Make sure the label bears 'noncomedogenic' or 'nonaknegenic' so that the product does not tend to block pores.

Don't: Pass the sunscreen, whether it's cloudy or cold outside (there is no reason) if you go to the beach or around a reflective surface like snow or ice, your skin foam with more sunscreen with a minimum SPF 30.

➢ You Are What You Eat.

Do: Notice what you place on your plate. Eat fresh, green, protein, and vitamin fruits. Diets that are rich in vitamin C and low-fat and sugar promote radiant skin. Consider a low-sugar diet, which can help cells maintain a healthy balance by lowering insulin levels.

"Don't: Eat spicy food and fermentation, salt, orange fruits, fried food. Instead of wanting a hot food like rice, oatmeal and apple", suggesting American writers and doctors Ayurvedic, Vasaved Lad, in the full book of Ayurvedic home medicine.

➢ Sweat!

Do it: Exercise always. Running, jogging will give your body the blood circulation needed and also speed up the process of cleaning your whole body. Will you see the light on your face after exercising and racing against time? Just walk fast around the block.

Do not: Skip skincare before and after practice. Before going out, use a toner to assist reduce oil production.

Exfoliation after, and then apply shea butter or olive oil to moisturize the skin.

Beauty tip for faces: 10 dos and a ban on beautiful skinny naturally is some brilliant beauty tips for the face to get the light you always want. Explore our beauty secrets, determine your skincare problems and follow our tricks regularly to get beautiful skin naturally.

➤ Beauty Sleep.

Do: Try to sleep a minimum of 8 hours every night. If you don't get enough to close your eyes, your skin is tired like you - it says, and you get a bag. So don't take risks. You can also use honey on your face twice or three times a week to naturally calm and heal your skin.

➤ H2O For Rescue.

Do Hydration yourself. Drink too much water every day, at least eight glasses, if not more. Also, eat fruits and vegetables that have high water content, such as watermelon, cucumber, orange, strawberries, Bali oranges, and cantaloupe. Ayurvedic Physician Vasant Lad recommends "Drinking water from a blue bottle" because it has a cooling effect.

Don't: Ignore roses. This helps prevent and reduce swelling in the morning, maintain a balance of pH and naturally hydrate your skin if you can prepare it during the day.

➢ Goodbye, Acne.

DO: Wash your face three times a day with warm water and gently massage it in a circular manner, making sure that the cleanser contains alpha hydroxy acid or beta hydroxy acids. Packages containing Multani face Mitti (Fuller's Earth) work very well too. After cleaning, Pat dry and apply a lotion containing benzoyl peroxide ", advises Dr. Zaheer Ahmed, Dokterologist, Max Hospitals. Benzoyl Peroxide is apparently effective for antibacterial action.

Do not: POP pimples because it can cause more swelling, redness, and even scarring. Feel acne is on his way? After cleaning the region with rose water, lay a cold green tea bag in the area for 10 minutes. Also, if you wear glasses or shades, wipe them regularly to prevent oil from clogging the pores around your eyes and nose.

➢ Return To Your Roots.

Do: Use a scrub Ayurvedic to nourish the skin and help better sip. Fortunately for you, all you need is already in your kitchen. 2 tbsp Chickpea flour, ½ tsp turmeric powder, a pinch of camphor, and sandalwood with rose water/milk/water is your skincare package which was perfect. Yes, the secret of beauty lies in the ancient Ayurveda.

Do not: ignore the basics. Sudarshan Kriya Mantra Create Your beauty. Yes, that's easy. Just breathing properly can eliminate freckles and acne. Nidhi Gureja, Living Arts, said, "Sudarshan Kriya is a breathing technique that incorporates specific natural rhythms of breath that harmonize the body, mind, and emotions. It helps release the accumulated stress, and the experience of each individual is different."

➢ Day Spa Every Day?

Do: Have a regular skincare regimen. "For dry skin, use a mask of fresh cherries. Apply a fresh cherry pulp on your face before going to bed. Let stand for 15 minutes and wash with lukewarm water," add the American writer Vasant Lad.

Do not: Forget to spoil yourself. A gentle facial massage with oil can work wonders. Depending on your skin type, choose from Mustard Oil, Coconut, Almond, or Kumkadi because they are an excellent nourishing agent that helps get a glowing complexion. Better yet - turn on some soothing instrumental music. After 20 minutes, what do you have? Your skin is beautiful and relaxing.

➢ Healthy Habits.

Do: Set aside time for you and strive to stay as stress-free as possible. Have you found that you tend to get out more when you're stressed? This is due to the fact that stress leads your body to create cortisol and other hormones, which causes your skin to become oilier. Stress management practices such as breathing exercises, yoga, and meditation should be practiced. The more you meditate, the more you emit.

Do not: Ignore the jaw and facial muscles. For just 5 minutes a day, do some facial exercises. You can just your bottom lip in such a way that the wrinkles created on the chin, then lower your chin to your chest. Another exercise that works awe is to look toward the ceiling and scowled. It stretches the muscles making the skin firmer.

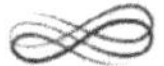

How Do You Look Beautiful Without Makeup?

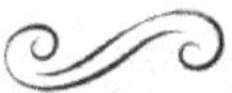

Frankly, this is all about your inside and how well you keep yourself. Yes! You must pay attention to important aspects of your diet, your habits, your lifestyle, and your skincare routine. If you even have one of these chaotic elements, the effect will definitely reflect your health and your overall appearance. Let's see the tips!

1.   Eat Your Way To Shine Skin.

A nutritious diet is an anti-stupid way to reach healthy skin. Make sure you receive your quotidian dose of fruits and veggies. Foods that are rich in omega-3 fatty acids such as flaxseed, walnuts, and food-enriched vitamins such as oranges, sweet potatoes, and pumpkins are a must. It also includes foods that are high protein, like eggs, chicken, kidney beans, lentils, beans, and cheese cottages. A healthy diet does your own work to make you shine and be healthy from the inside by giving your body everything you need.

2.   Drink Lots Of Water.

We cannot simply emphasize the main of H2O. Every system and purpose in our body depends on water. Drinking at least eight or more glasses helps remove toxins from your body, and hence your skin looks fat and more alive. It also helps maintain wrinkles in the bay.

The best way to ingest water is to fill bottles with cucumbers, lemon, zucchinis, mint leaves, and other brightly colored vegetables and make detox water you drink while traveling. Doing this gives you nutrition and hydration to help your body utilize and hold water more efficiently.

3.   Sleep Peacefully.

Sleep sounds run along with your appearance and feel. It's important because your body fixes itself when you sleep. Just like you need to charge your cellphone, your body needs to fill yourself and live a day with your battery at 50 percent, which only leads to extra tension and inefficiencies. 6-8 hours of sleep quality is very important for you to wake up feeling and look great. By doing this, you will have an enthusiastic pattern, less than the black circle feared under your eyes, and you will slow down your aging process. The skin produces a new tendon when you sleep. Don't let anything in the world avert you and beauty you sleep!

4.   Become Aware Of The Material.

Beauty that is aware of material is something. Yes! Just like what you put in your body affects your overall health, what you put on the same surface. Your skin absorbs 60 percent of the items you use, so make sure you do research on the materials present in skincare, hair care, and your beauty products. Keep away from services that contain parabens, petrochemicals, and sulfates that can cause irritation to your skin or make your hair dry and frizzy. The best thing is to stick to products that contain natural ingredients.

5.   Working With Healthy Skin.

Physical activity is very important, both for your physical and mental health. Do something - anything jams - whether it's about the gym, running, doing yoga, or going swimming. Scientifically proven exercises take advantage of your skin and improve your mood. A base of three hours per week of physical activity will result in an increase in your health. It improves your blood circulation, helps eliminate toxins, increases the amount of oxygen delivered to your skin, giving a boost of endorphins that reduce stress and soothe your whole body, including your skin! However, if you're title to the park for a run, do not forget to wear sunscreen.

6.   Stick For A Consistent Skin Of Routine Maintenance.

You want to know your skin type and find a skincare routine that works for you. CTM is routinely cleaning, tightening, and moisturizing, which is important for skin health. The type of product you use to follow this method is entirely dependent on your skin type. Follow the morning and consistent night routine, and we guarantee that you will see a drastic increase in the appearance of your skin. Also, don't, in any circumstances, go to bed without cleaning it. You will only invite a number of problems for your skin. Use hand cream and body lamb for hands and feet.

7. Exfoliation Is Key.

Make exfoliating the skin an important part of your skincare regime. This is indeed the key to bright skin. Your skin always spills dead cells from the surface that helps to renew itself with fresh and healthy cells. Give this natural process help with a light exfoliator. The advantages of dead cells sitting on the surface of your skin can cause stuffers of pores, blackheads, acne, and acne. If you instill exfoliating skin into your regime, serum and moisturizer are better absorbed into the skin, making them work more efficiently. Choose a soft scrub or make a natural scrub itself at home using ingredients such as gram flour or coffee scrub. Maintain skin peel a maximum of twice a week. You will see improvements seen in your skin health - it will look fresher and smoother.

8. Make A Mandatory Sunscreen.

Sunscreen is not an option. UVA the Sun, UVB, and UVC Sinar are the main causes of premature aging on the skin. If you go after this one easy step, you will thank yourself in the future. This helps prevent dark spots and hyper-pigmentation. The SPF, which is the 'Sun Protection Factor, determines how well the sunscreen will protect you. Dermatologists recommend that you use a minimum of SPF 30 before stepping out.

9.   Stress Breasts.

We all have insane schedules in today's contemporary society, and stress is unavoidable. Uncontrolled stress, on the other hand, can lead to headaches and hypertension. It can also cause acne, hair loss, and gray hair. This is only a severe result of a few stresses. So, while you can't fully avoid the bill, work, your life, and all the stress that comes with it, you have to find a way to manage it. Meditate, drink a nice cup of tea, listen to music or make some time for whatever you love. Do take cold pills now and then!

10. Drink Green Tea.

There is a reason why green tea is very popular among health fans. This is probably a healthy drink out there and enriched with nutrients and antioxidants that are very beneficial for the body. It contains 'catechins,' which is an antioxidant form that prevents cell damage. This increases blood circulation, cholesterol, lowers and blood pressure, and improves your skin health. The EGCG material present in this tea also helps in weight loss by reducing fat absorption. Get used to brewing yourself some green tea!

11.   Give Your Face A Massage.

This is a secret skin DIY professionals swear by. A good face massage every day can reduce the appearance of fine lines, tighten the skin and make it look more radiant. Besides that, it also makes you feel relieved from stress and rejuvenate. This procedure is used in China to target certain pressure areas on the face. When massaging your skin, you might apply lotion or coconut oil to keep it moisturized.

12. Pamper Tress You.

Have you ever imagined all the sweat, pollution, and dirt that make your hair of natural light? Soft and glossy hair is a sign of healthy hair. It's important to take care of your keys by providing food for your hair. You can achieve this by oiling your hair at least once a week with coconut, olive, or almond oil. Hair spa treatment is also important as oiling does not provide enough food. Use hair services that are free of sulfates and other damaging chemicals. Avoid using hotness on your hair and try to leave it in its natural state as often as possible without the need to remove hair styling tools that only temporarily damage your hair looks good. Invest in a good rest or serum enriched with the goodness of the Moroccan Argan oil instead. Naturally, shiny hair only adds to your beauty.

13. Wear Clothes That Fit.

What you wear influences how you present yourself. Make sure all of your clothes fit you perfectly. Stock your wardrobe with clothes that compliment you and look flattering on your figure. Wearing clothes that are too tight or too loose can be uncomfortable and can add excess body. Clothing that does not fit you well just ruins your style. Add some extra effort to find things when you shop. It makes your body look flatter and also allows you to breathe.

14.   Act Sweet Well.

Nourishing yourself from head to toe is very important for your appearance. Is not it also felt good to take care of each of you as a whole? Pamper yourself a little and at the salon for a mani-pedi and a facial at the weekend. Also, it is important to keep your current eyebrows framing your face, and we cannot stress enough the significance of the large brow. Make appointments for regular wax and remove excess hair (if this is important to you). Overall, fixed Kempati every day - to bathe regularly, use perfumes or deodorants, hair care for you, and keep you clean.

15.   Keep Your Smile.

Your pearly whites are in need of maintenance and health of your mouth to talk about you. Visit your dentist every six months or so and follow a regular routine as brushing your teeth at least twice a day with fluoride toothpaste is good. Floss on a daily basis, use mouthwash and maintain a healthy, clean grin. Select the appropriate toothbrush and clean your teeth in the proper manner: up and down in a slightly circular motion. Bestow a great smile so much to gain and also boost your confidence to a completely new level!

16.   Get Regular Hair Trim.

Getting regular trims enhances the look and feel of your hair. Make sure you get your hair cut on a regular basis (at least once in two months). By cutting the ends that are not healthy, your hair will have damage and flyaway lower, adding volume and shine. If you want to grow your hair, the trim is recommended for healthy hair growth faster.

17. Dealing With Pesky Acne The Right Way.

Breakout is natural, and everyone had to go through this ordeal - some more than others. However, there is no need to worry. Let me tell you, the defeat thing you can do for your new friend is tried to get rid of him appear. Do not, under any circumstances, touch your pimples or try to blackmail - you will only make the situation worse. Instead, choose a method that will treat the pesky baby and escape without leaving a scar. You can put some tea tree oil on the zit and be patient until it dries. You can also use benzoyl peroxide to get rid of it. Use a face wash with salicylic acid percentage, and you can avoid breakouts for most. Patience is the key here!

18. Use Basic Food Supplements.

A healthy diet is very vital, but sometimes, we lose a lot of nutrients because they are not part of our diet. Please note that you cannot take this supplement instead of ordinary food and survive, but you can add this to your diet plan to increase its benefits. Popular supplements include vitamins A, B12, C, D, and E, calcium and iron, zinc, and special products such as fish oil and probiotics. Health supplements are very important because factors such as alcohol, infection, and allergies quickly drain their nutritional body.

19. Cut Junk.

'Trash' here refers to various items such as foods that are unhealthy, alcohol, cigarettes, and all other garbage consumed without thinking. Put full of fast food like burgers, fries, soda, and other fried sweet items will make a big difference in your health and overall appearance. It is also best to reduce excess sugar, alcohol, and smoking because they are not only dangerous for your vital organs, but this is also a factor that leads to other problems that clearly show your appearance. So cut it all and maintain a good balance between healthy food and fast food.

20. Invest In A Night Cream.

The night cream will help you wake up the best. Many of you might ask if night cream is needed, and the answer is great! During the day, we are all revealed to pollution, smoke, sun, and many free radicals that emphasize our skin and cause premature aging. You need to take advantage of the night to rejuvenate your skin by providing enough nutrition and moisture. You should consider investing in high-quality night creams that fit your skin type when your skin is in rest mode and repair. Getting a good night to relax with a night cream will drastically change the way your skin looks and feels in the morning!

21. Maintain Good Posture.

The right posture alignment will not only allow you to work more efficiently and avoid tension in your spine, muscles, and ligaments but also affect how you release the people around you. Bad wrap and posture can make you look older than damage your back, and have a negative impact on your energy level. Always pay attention to how you sit, walk and move as this is really important - even when you get older.

22. Whip Up Some DIY Face Masks.

What's better than pampering myself on Friday night with a nutritious face mask? It sounds relaxed, right? It's easy to make these masks in the comfort of your home with ingredients from your kitchen (if you like to keep it natural). Routine weekly masks help your skin get extra attention and attention, let it energize and rejuvenate. Based on your skin type, arrange a mask that suits your needs, place it and relax! You can use ingredients such as honey, aloe vera, gram flour, yogurt, oatmeal, and fruits because these are some very popular choices for homemade masks.

23. Sleep On A Silk Pillowcase.

Sleeping in silk pillowcases is great for your face and hair - it can help them stay healthy and smooth and can reduce the appearance of fine lines and wrinkles on your face. Silk also resists dust mites and other allergens naturally. This pillowcase has become a new FAD, but besides its just FAD, they have some very substantial benefits. You need to try it to believe it!

24. Engage In Activities That Make You Happy.

In addition to all external factors, the most important thing is to be truly happy. Stress and monotonous daily life hurt our sparks and make us depressed and sad. Take the time to do some fun activities such as painting, cycling, listening to music, and cooking, even though the only thing that makes you happy is making your morning coffee alive for the enjoyment of coffee and making it extraordinary. Take the time to aim for the magical part of happiness and life. It has to do with making your soul happy!

25. Strive For Yourself, Lack And All.

You need to love yourself to the point that your energy and aura reject anyone who doesn't know your value. Self-love is not selfish; This is as important as the love you give to others. We all have shortcomings, but if you cancel the shortcomings - it means rejecting your entire lump without you won't be you. We don't preach here but only give some suggestions - embracing every bit of you!

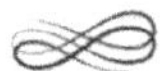

Natural Ways To Have Beautiful And Young Skin

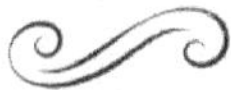

Do not smoke. Sleep soundly. Often exercise. Stay out of the sun—loading antioxidants. Eat organic food.

We know. We have heard everything before. We know how to keep young skin ... or whether we have to get out of the sun and chew blueberries, there are many more things you can do to ensure that your skin remains clear, smooth, and durable when you press an age where wrinkles and Age spots should be part of your life.

Some of the following 10 secrets may surprise you:

1.   Drink Lots Of Water.

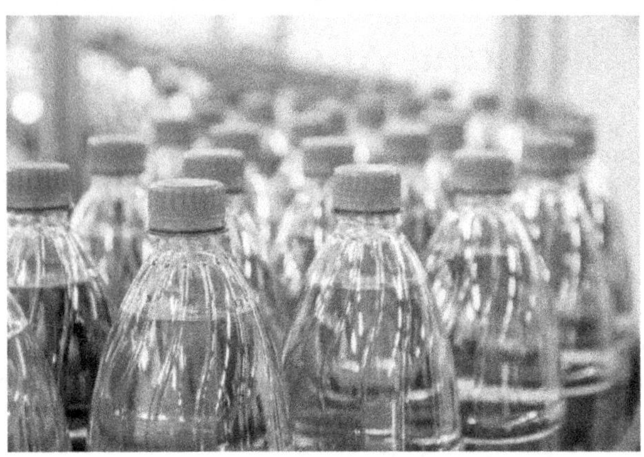

If you have time, see Christie Brinkley.

So, what is the secret? Water. During the days of modeling, he drank at least one liter of water a day, which was a smart step. Because water evaporates from the skin, you need to continue to fill your body with water. If not, your skin will dry and saggy. Water keeps your skin plump, elastic, and smooth. So skip coke and fit in H2O. Your future yourself will be grateful.

2.   Eat Cooked Tomatoes.

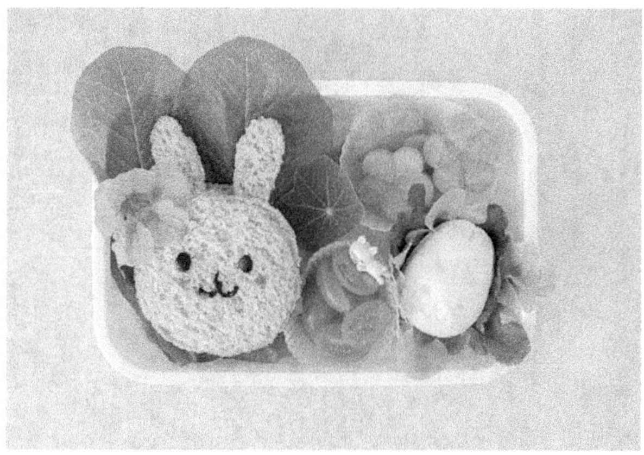

Yes, you read it correctly. Cooked tomatoes are one of the best meals you can eat to keep young skin. Tomatoes are full of strong antioxidants called lycopene, which helps protect the skin from sun damage. Lycopene is best absorbed by the body when cooked or processed, therefore cooked tomatoes. In this case, choose some grilled tomatoes, tomato sauce, tomato paste, or organic soy sauce, not raw tomatoes.

3. Eat Red Meat.

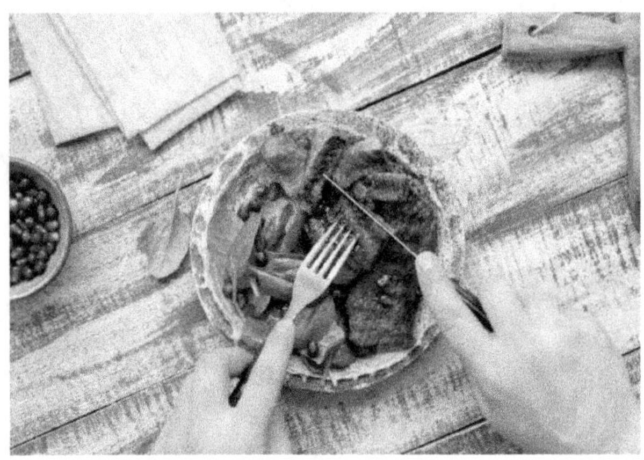

Red meat gets a lot of leaves because it's fatty, bad for the heart, and is full of hormones. All that might be true, but if you want young skin, you better start preparing steaks.

When drunk in a medium number, red meat is actually good for the skin because it is loaded with protein and zinc. It was also found to treat acne better than antibiotics. Proteins found in meat contain high concentrations of amino acids (proline and glycine, for specific) your body needs to produce collagen. Zinc is also just what doctor-erordered dermatologists because it produces a lot of collagen and has anti-inflammatory properties.

If you don't eat red meat, all hopes are not lost. There are many foods that increase other collagen that you can load, such as fruit, soybeans, oranges, nuts, and eggs.

4.   Develop An Addiction To Green Tea.

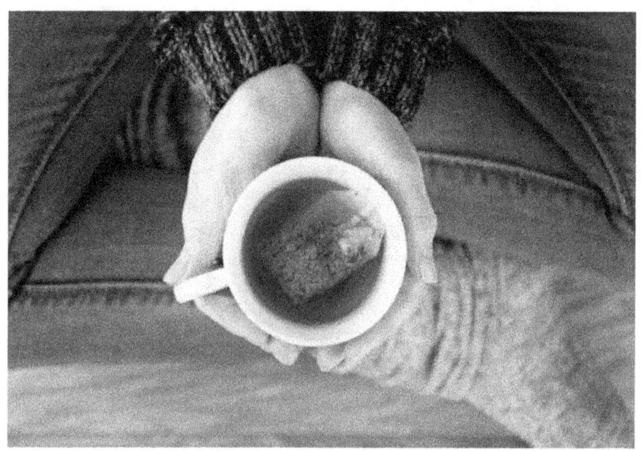

Everyone and their mothers know that green tea is full of antioxidants, but who doesn't everyone know is that drinking a cup of green tea twice a day for six months can actually reverse the damage to sunlight on your skin.

Green tea has a tall concentration of catechins, antioxidants that are famous for their anti-aging effects. This protects your skin against UV radiation, so it helps prevent the growth of moles and age spots. Catching also has several anti-inflammatory powers that help delay wrinkles.

5.   Or Go For White Tea.

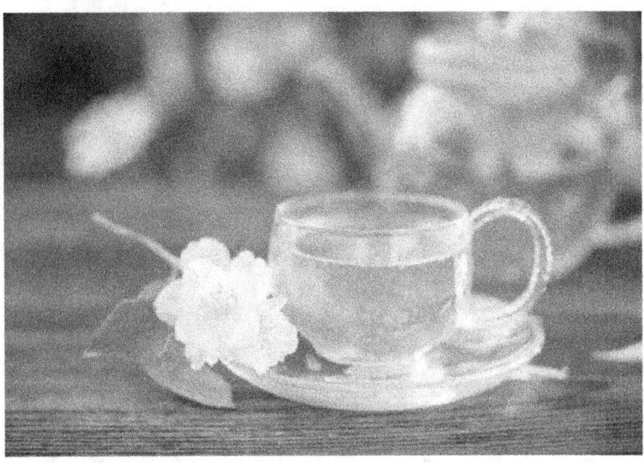

If green tea is not your teacup (sorry, can't refuse), then consider taking a cup of white tea. It does not provide the same benefits as green tea, but useful. White tea's anti-aging qualities protect collagen and other structural proteins in the skin. This prevents enzyme activity that breaks down collagen and causes wrinkles.

6. Snacks On Carrots.

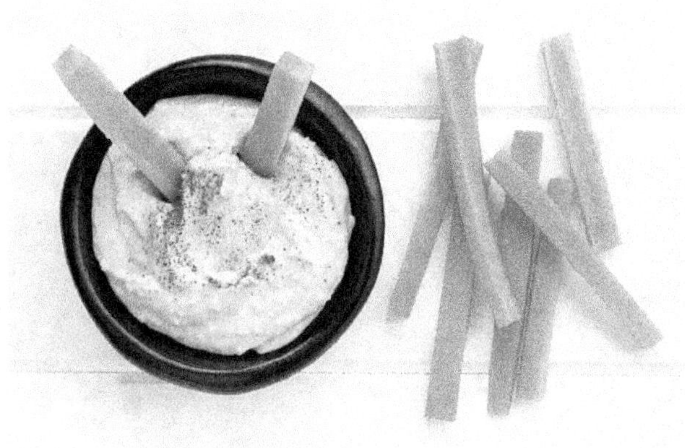

If you want smooth, beautiful, young skin, you need a healthy dose of vitamin A every day. Look no further than orange vegetables, such as carrots and sweet potatoes, because they are rich in vitamin A and will help restore and regenerate damaged collagen.

7.   Choose Natural Skincare Products.

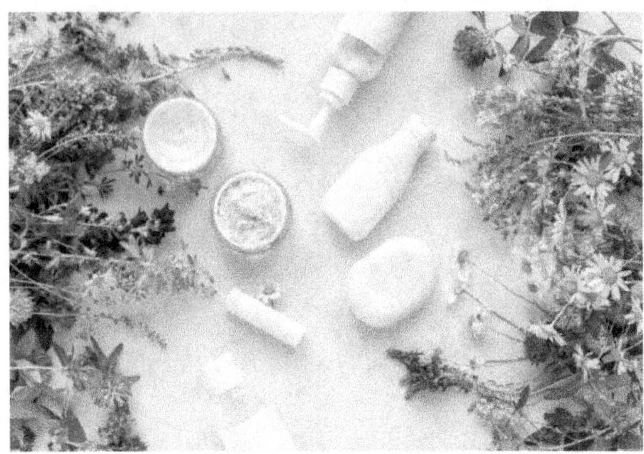

Many skincare products are loaded with harsh chemicals that will actually accelerate the aging process of your skin. You better use natural skin care products because they contain properties that are derived from plants. However, you should constantly verify the contents to guarantee that the items you intend to buy will improve your skin.

8.   Avoid Toxic Cleaning Products.

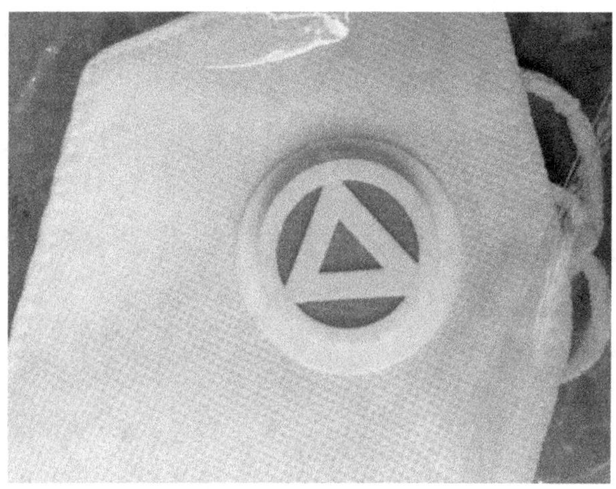

What is the relationship between cleaning products with wrinkles? A lot, actually. Your skin absorbs toxic chemicals (which often happens when you spray the cleaning product on the surface), and it accelerates the aging process of your skin.

9. Wash Your Face With Honey.

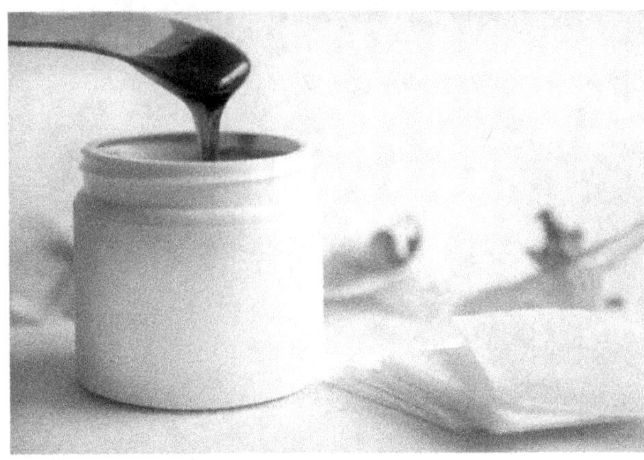

Did you know that Cleopatra took a bath of milk and honey to keep her skin fresh and wrinkle-free? He's on to something because honey is fantastic for your skin. It is full of antioxidants, opens your pores, and moisturizes your skin. So ditch the washing of the face (which may be loaded with harsh chemicals) and begin washing the face with honey!

10. Turmeric Menyeser All Over Your Face.

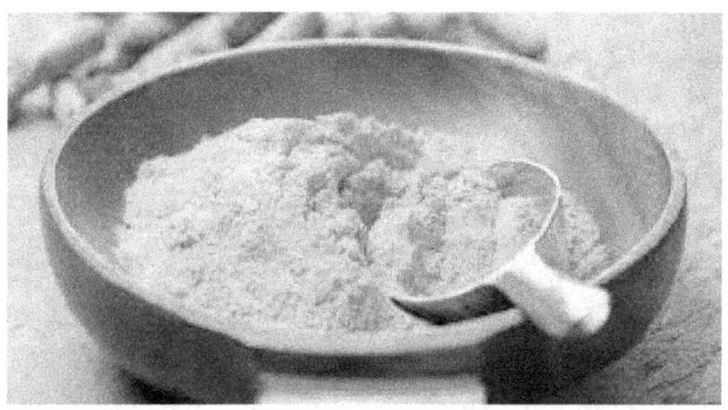

They have done something right because the anti-inflammatory properties of turmeric soften the skin, clear acne, reduce inflammation, and reduce wrinkles.

So, how exactly do you make a mess all over your face? Of course, by applying turmeric face mask! Here's how to go about it:

Mix together:
- One teaspoon ground turmeric
- rice flour (two teaspoons) (for oily skin) or oats that have been finely ground (for dry or mature skin)
- plain yogurt (three tablespoons) (or milk, cream, or sour cream)
- Applying the mixture on your clean face, and then let it dry. After 15-20 minutes, rinse. Try to do this once a week, and if it goes well, increase the frequency every day or every day.

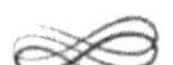

Drug Houses Favorite For Younger-Looking Skin

Finding fair skincare to look younger does not need a magic potion or a trip to the drug store. You can get younger-looking skin by using a few basic ingredients from your kitchen and making some small changes in your daily routine. The sooner you apply this home remedy, the easier it is to prevent damage to the skin and reduce the signs of aging. Think of it as your future share some smart skincare tips with your younger self.

Which one works for you? Select your secret tricks for younger-looking skin.

1. Crack Open The Coconut Oil.

Coconut oil is a usual ingredient in many skincare products but can be used alone to create younger-looking skin. Non-greasy moisturizer can be applied every day to your face or your entire body. His wealth makes it a great moisturizer overnight, but it works fine any time of day. Be sure to look for the quality of liquid coconut oil cold didekatan. As a bonus, it has antimicrobial goods that protect the skin from infection.

2.   Craft Your Own Toner.

Press the right tone with toner DIY you can make at home. Toner helps control oil and freshen your skin's protective layer. You can set up your own batch by using a combination of cooling peppermint, sage, and witch hazel. Add one teaspoon of sage leaves and a teaspoon of peppermint leaves to four ounces of witch hazel. Steep for three days and then rub into your skin with a cotton ball.

3.   Heal The Skin With Honey.

Sweetheart is rich in nutrients and is a great moisturizer for skin of all ages. It also helps speed up the regeneration of cells and can even reduce the appearance of wrinkles when used regularly. You can just slather honey on the face and neck, then rinse with warm water after 20 minutes. For extra light, mix 2 tablespoons of honey with milk powder and water to create a mask that softens your skin and helps lighten dark spots.

4.   Along Your Skin With Lemon.

Don't let dark spots and agenda skin ensure your appearance. Use astringent lemon properties to relieve skin spots and age. Lemon spends your skin tone and brightens your skin. There is no special recipe, simply give a little lemon juice on the cotton ball and apply it to your skin every day as a refreshing toner. In the morning, squeeze a lemon into hot or cold water to stimulate the entire body.

5. Keep Reddish Skin With Roses.

What is the most recommended house remedies material? Rave skincare experts about combinations of roses, rice powder, and milk. Combine these three super foods to make a thick paste, then apply to your face and set aside for 20 minutes. Rosewater brightens the appearance of your skin, and rice helps your skin produces more collagen to increase elasticity, and the milk is soothing to lighten the dark area of the skin. Plus, this skincare home medicine feels fancy and smells fantastic.

6. Fix The Skin Overnight.

Whatever skincare drug you choose, use it overnight. When you sleep, skin cells are busy updating themselves and repairing damage from that day. Help them by making sure they have natural ingredients and moisturize that speed up the process. The homemade overnight face mask will have a more durable effect than you just use in the bathroom. Don't forget to treat your lips for eight hours of hydration by wearing a lip balm before going to bed.

7. Bathing Is Strategically.

A warm shower helps cure your skin by opening the pores and releasing poisons. But using too much time in a hot water shower can remove oil to hydrate your skin and cause drought. It's best to keep your hot shower short and lower the temperature if it's comfortable. For extra encouragement, give your skin a cold water explosion at the end of your bathroom. This helps improve circulation and can enlighten dull skin tones.

8. Try Tomatoes.

Next time you are on the market, take a few tomatoes for a refreshing face mask. Place the tomato slices on your face for 20 minutes to rejuvenate stressful skin, tired. Tomatoes help reduce inflammation and naturally brighten the skin. If you feel silly sitting with tomato slices on your face, you can also combine tomato porridge with olive oil to make a smooth, delicious face mask).

9. Moisturize After Being Washed.

This easy skincare practice is important to add to your routine, especially if your skin is dry. It also helps you maintain a youthful appearance all over your body. When you dry your skin after washing your face, leave it a little moist. Then apply the moisturizer or body oil to lock the moisture so that your skin is hydrated deeper and maintain a young and attentive look.

10. Use Sugar In The Right Way.

Sugar has the upper side and downside to keep the skin looking younger. The disadvantage is that eating a lot of sugar can cause blood sugar nails, triggering insulin release, which causes inflammation in your skin. Reducing sugar will keep the skin feeling tight and healthy. The side of sugar is that it is a great exfoliation. Create a simple face scrub by combining sugar and olive oil in a container that you can save in your shower or in the sink.

11.   Switch Your Sleep Routine.

Don't worry, and you don't need to change what time you go to bed, just by the way you sleep. Experts endorse sleeping on your back so your pillows don't add wrinkles to your skin all night. If you have to sleep in your stomach or side, change the side of your face you sleep. Also, increasing your pillowcase to a softer sateen or silk fabric will be less abrasive for your face and keep your skin looking younger.

12.   Humidify Your Home.

Take care of your skin soft and young by adding a moisturizer to your home. Make sure you place one in your room, so you can get at least eight hours of additional moisture. You might also want to add a humidifier to another room where you spend a lot of time, like a den or your head office. They are great for winter when the air outside is dry, and a humidifier also helps in the summer because the air conditioner removes moisture from the air.

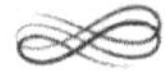

Ways To Maintain A Youthful Appearance

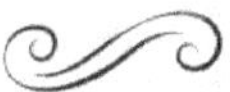

> ### Stay Out Of The Sun.

Although it is true that the sun is not the only factor in the overall appearance of your skin, it does play a big role. In fact, damage from UV sunlight (UVA and UVB rays) is responsible for around 90% of the signs of aging your skin seen. UV light breaks the elastin on your skin, causing a sagging and dull appearance, wrinkles, age spots, uneven skin tones, and more.

Always (always, always, always) wear a quality sunscreen with a minimum SPF ranking of 30, and make sure it is a broad-spectrum sunscreen - which means blocking UVA and UVB rays. Keep in mind that sunlight comes out whether it's bright or not, so make sure you use sunscreen every day. And remember to re-register every few hours for maximum protection.

> ### Drink Lots Of Water.

Another key for the skin to look younger is hydration. You must aim for 8 cups of water filtered every day to keep your skin looking radiant and support optimal health. Dehydration can quickly cause your skin to look dry and dull - emphasizing wrinkles and aging. Drink enough water every day to refill your network and cell skin, allowing younger and healthier skin.

➢ Get ZZZ.

Another key to maintaining a young appearance is to just rest! When you sleep, your body continues to issue a hormone that promotes cell turnover and updates. Use this time for your advantage - this is when you have to use challenging activation of age such as retinoid and beta hydroxy acid, which is strong exfoliates and wrinkle eraser. But keep in mind that this grows your sensitivity to sunlight, so be extra alert with sunscreen.

To take further steps, consider increasing the satin pillowcase. Over time, throw and turn on a fabric that is rougher, like cotton, which can contribute to collagen damage in your skin, which leads to wrinkles.

➢ Rub.

While water keeps your skin moisturized from the inside out, you can also aid him by using the correct moisturizer on a regular basis. Hydrated skin does not only look better, but it is also stronger and more capable of fighting irritation. Moisturizer consists of two components to help your skin feel soft and chewy: Humektan, which draws water from the air to your skin, and Emollients, which help strengthen the lipid barrier of your skin and hold moisture. Creams and moisturizers are not all made the same. It is important to use clinical class products with better absorption and penetration into the skin, also with higher active ingredients, for best results, and supported by clinical studies that are proven to treat and protect the skin. These results are driven by clinical skincare products only sold in medical practices like us.

➢ Eat A Rich Plant Diet.

The benefits of a heavy diet in many fruits and vegetables. They provide major nutrients that help support healthy aging and keep your body young, both inside and outside. Fruits and vegetables also increase your phytonutrient intake, which helps your body ward off the effects of damaging free radicals found in the environment—aiming to eat a healthy diet consisting of mostly fruits and vegetables, coupled with grains and healthy, lean protein.

➢ Get.

Stay active is very helpful in maintaining a healthy weight, but do you know that it has also been proven to help you look younger? Research has shown that strengthening exercises, especially high-intensity interval training (HIIT), can slow your aging at a cellular level of almost 10 years. But the benefits do not stop there - sports also increase blood flow, moving oxygen and critical nutrients throughout your body, which leads to a younger appearance. Furthermore, regular exercise is very important to maintain strength and muscle mass, which also offers a lot of health benefits and can add a year to your life.

➤ Build A Good Routine.

Even though there are steps that can be taken to help reverse damage to your skin, it is much easier to help prevent damage before it starts. Create a good skincare routine for your daily habits. Aim to use a soft and exfoliate cleaner, and make sure you use the right care and serum for your type and skin needs. And make sure to use the daily moisturizer to increase your skin elasticity and stay hydrated.

➤ Limit Alcohol And Caffeine.

While we like the good martini or latte as much as the next, and alcohol and caffeine can have health benefits when consumed in moderate quantities, too much can bring havoc on your skin. Both can dehydrate your body and rob the main nutrients. The worse is that some of these effects can be permanent.

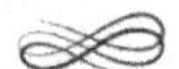

Refrence And Citation

1. https://www.townandcountrymag.com/style/beauty-products/g19410418/how-to-look-younger/

2. https://www.everydayhealth.com/pictures/look-younger-now/

3. https://www.pureluxemedical.com/blog/8-ways-to-maintain-a-youthful-appearance

4. https://www.ditchthelabel.org/15-beauty-tips-for-teens/?gclid=Cj0KCQiA7oyNBhDiARIsADtGRZY 8lFIiyYΛ925SP7UyqpXpTBnyfkh7tliAZvoFcQgAc GNXh8T-P5T4aAu3LEALw_wcB

5. https://www.mindbodygreen.com/0-8355/15-natural-ways-to-maintain-beautiful-youthful-skin.html

6. https://www.mindbodygreen.com/0-8355/15-natural-ways-to-maintain-beautiful-youthful-skin.html

7. https://kidshealth.org/en/teens/skin-tips.html

8. https://pharmeasy.in/blog/simple-home-remedies-for-glowing-skin/

9. https://www.beautifulhameshablog.com/glowing-skin-for-teenagers-best-tips-and-home-remedies/

10. https://www.workitdaily.com/beauty-therapy-courses

11. https://www.staceyjamesinstitute.com/benefits-of-attending-beauty-courses/

12. https://beautifultouches.com/15-subtle-ways-to-enhance-your-natural-beauty/

13. https://www.belfasttelegraph.co.uk/life/fashion-beauty/10-simple-tips-to-enhance-your-natural-beauty-29041319.html

14. https://www.wikihow.com/Enhance-Your-Beauty-and-Looks

15. https://www.belfasttelegraph.co.uk/life/fashion-beauty/10-simple-tips-to-enhance-your-natural-beauty-29041319.html

16. https://www.femina.in/beauty/skin/how-to-enhance-your-natural-beauty-189308.html

17. https://www.glamour.com/story/free-diy-beauty-hacks-for-clear-skin

18. https://greatist.com/health/home-remedies-for-glowing-skin

19. https://www.indiatvnews.com/lifestyle/beauty-skin-care-tips-7-effective-home-remedies-for-healthy-and-flawless-skin-466671

20. https://www.indiatvnews.com/lifestyle/beauty-skin-care-tips-7-effective-home-remedies-for-healthy-and-flawless-skin-466671

21. https://www.everydayhealth.com/skin-beauty/10-best-natural-clear-skin-remedies/

22. https://themasking.com/skincare-tips-10-dos-and-donts-for-naturally-beautiful-skin/

23. https://timesofindia.indiatimes.com/life-style/beauty/dos-and-donts-for-naturally-glowing-skin/articleshow/16912892.cms

24. https://www.spagregories.com/beauty-tips-for-face-7-dos-and-donts-for-naturally-beautiful-skin/

25. https://www.purecosmetics.info/face-care-tips/

26. https://food.ndtv.com/beauty/how-to-look-beautiful-without-makeup-1224170

27. https://timesofindia.indiatimes.com/life-style/beauty/skin-care-12-natural-ways-to-look-beautiful-without-makeup/articleshow/83600421.cms

28. https://www.wikihow.com/Look-Good-Without-Makeup

29. https://timesofindia.indiatimes.com/life-style/beauty/skin-care-12-natural-ways-to-look-beautiful-without-makeup/articleshow/83600421.cms

30. https://brightside.me/inspiration-girls-stuff/10-simple-rules-for-looking-great-without-makeup-292560/

31. https://viomedspa.com/six-ways-to-maintain-a-youthful-appearance/

32. https://www.hindustantimes.com/fashion-and-trends/how-to-look-young-these-20-natural-anti-ageing-tips-will-make-you-fall-in-love-with-yourself/story-5n5rVkbKh2KJBlFQoLz6bI.html

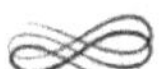

9 789392 878862